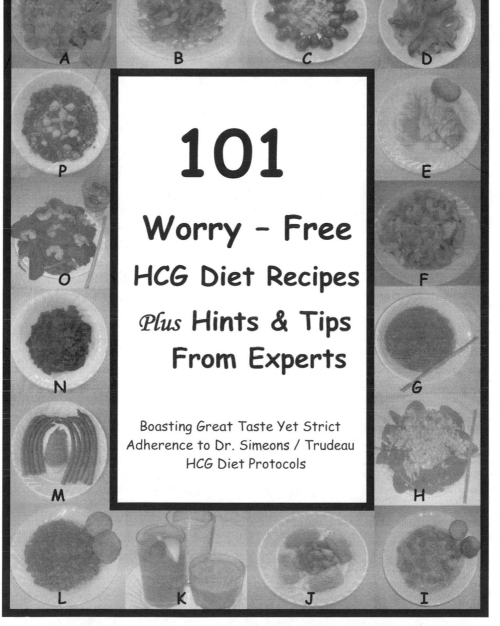

101

Worry – Free
HCG Diet Recipes
Plus Hints & Tips
From Experts

Boasting Great Taste Yet Strict
Adherence to Dr. Simeons / Trudeau
HCG Diet Protocols

For the most comprehensive, step-by-step guide to maximizing your HCG weight loss success obtain the:

HCG Weight Loss Cure Guide

A Supplemental Guide to Dr. Simeons' Pounds and Inches as referenced in Kevin Trudeau's The Weight Loss Cure "They" Don't Want You to Know About
A STEP BY STEP GUIDE TO MAXIMIZING YOUR HCG WEIGHT LOSS SUCCESS

in hard copy from CreateSpace (the publisher) on Amazon.com OR, for instant availability, the pdf format from www.hcgweightlosscureguide.com or www.poundsandinchesaway.com.

Table of Contents

Dedication

This book is dedicated to all the HCG dieters who have complained about boredom with the food choices Dr. Simeons so carefully selected, based on nutritional value and weight loss compatibility. We have indeed created a 'little book', as Dr. Simeons complains, but have taken special care to not count calories or otherwise contradict the intent of the diet. We have also taken special care to honor all aspects of the HCG diet while attempting to provide some variety and time-saving qualities for HCG participants who have limited time and/or cooking abilities. While we did not have boredom issues during our initial HCG cycle, we have certainly used many of these recipes since writing this book because these recipes are surprisingly tasty.

Enjoy!

Leanne and Linda

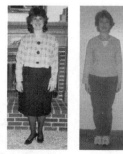 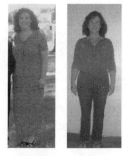

Before and After Pictures

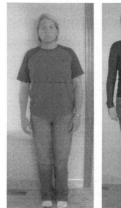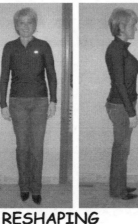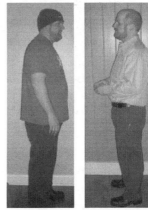

RESHAPING
2 rounds (only about 20 pounds)…almost unrecognizable!

40 pounds in 1 round

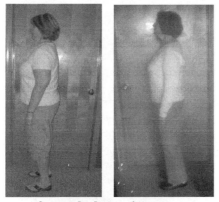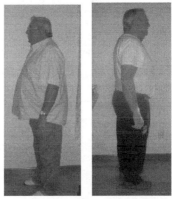

2 rounds down; 1 to go

2 Rounds – 60 pounds and holding

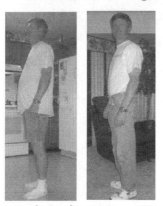

These results **ARE** typical.

Almost anyone will lose 20–30 pounds in a complete cycle if the diet is followed with recipes like those listed in this book. This is just a sampling of the successes we see on a weekly basis.

25 pounds in the minimum 23 days

Congratulations to all losers!

500 Calorie Diet (Phase 2 as referenced in Trudeau's book)
Following is the diet directly from Dr. Simeons' Manuscript:

The Diet

The 500 calorie diet is explained on the day of the second injection to those patients who will be preparing their own food, and it is most important that the person who will actually cook is present - the wife, the mother or the cook, as the case may be. Here in Italy patients are given the following diet sheet.

Breakfast: Tea or coffee in any quantity without sugar. Only one tablespoonful of milk allowed in 24 hours. Saccharin or Stevia may be used.

Lunch:
1. 100 grams of veal, beef, chicken breast, fresh white fish, lobster, crab, or shrimp. All visible fat must be carefully removed before cooking, and the meat must be weighed raw. It must be boiled or grilled without additional fat. Salmon, eel, tuna, herring, dried or pickled fish are not allowed. The chicken breast must be removed from the bird.
2. One type of vegetable only to be chosen from the following: spinach, chard, chicory, beet-greens, green salad, tomatoes, celery, fennel, onions, red radishes, cucumbers, asparagus, cabbage.
3. One breadstick (grissino) or one Melba toast.
4. An apple or a handful of strawberries or one-half grapefruit, orange* (*in the original manuscript, but not in at least one version of the circulating manuscripts)

Dinner : The same four choices as lunch.

The juice of one lemon daily is allowed for all purposes. Salt, pepper, vinegar, mustard powder, garlic, sweet basil, parsley, thyme, marjoram, etc., may be used for seasoning, but no oil, butter or dressing.

Tea, coffee, plain water, or mineral water are the only drinks allowed, but they may be taken in any quantity and at all times.

In fact, the patient should drink about 2 liters of these fluids per day.

Above Excerpt directly from Pounds and Inches: A New Approach to Obesity although a few mistakes have been corrected for ease of understanding.

Stevia

The thing about stevia …some people love it; some people have no use for it.

Health professionals have been telling us for years that saccharin (Sweet 'N Low), sucralose (Splenda), and aspartame (NutraSweet and Equal) are seriously toxic for us. Stevia is a natural sweetener that has been around for centuries. For more information on stevia, www.stevia.com is a good resource. A general search online will provide countless sites to satisfy your curiosity about stevia. Many provide an area for recipes, ordering, and other information.

Local stores are starting to carry stevia, but it may not be obvious without looking in the small print. For example, Schnucks Markets carry Only Sweet with 'Stevia Extract' in small letters under the product name.

I have, and use, Stevia on a daily basis and in all forms: liquid, packet, bulk. I have all 12 liquid flavors. I carry packets (in my purse, diaper bag, briefcase, and kitchen cabinet). I use the bulk shake form for cooking because it is less expensive per serving than the packets. Finally I have the liquid travel pack (4 flavors) in my purse. I use stevia, both when I am doing an HCG protocol and when I am not, for coffee, tea, water, raw food and cooked food – you might be surprised at how many seasoning spices have sugar in them.

Now, when you try recipes that call for stevia, be prepared to start out with the least amount and increase as necessary. We have experimented to derive these recipes, but your taste could be different, so play with stevia and fine tune the recipes to meet your taste buds' desires.

P.S. Per Dr. Simeons, saccharin and stevia are allowed on the 500 calorie diet phase of the HCG protocol. ZSweet, Lakanto and other 0 Calorie, alcohol sweeteners have carbohydrates and, therefore, we do NOT recommend those sweeteners while on the 500 calorie diet phase.

HCG Dieters Beware...

Spices, the unsuspected pitfall!

Sugar, in one form or another, is added to more food products, including spices and seasonings, than you can imagine. One would think that a few granules of sugar, when added to a person's diet, couldn't possibly make a difference, especially if the **Nutrition Facts Table** says **CALORIES 0, SUGARS 0**. This, however, is not the case. We have seen many people with slowed or even stalled weight loss due to the spices they were sprinkling on their food. There are two important points that must be understood.

First, according to nutrition labeling regulations, a **Nutrition Facts Table** must list the content of calories and 13 core nutrients per serving on most pre-packaged foods. The core nutrients include the total amount of **CARBOHYDRATE** and two types of carbohydrate in particular, **SUGARS** and **FIBER**. According to the regulation, a product can boast of '0 SUGAR' as long as it "contains < .5g sugars per reference amount and "free of energy" (< 5 cal per reference amount)." This means that a manufacturer can decide just how much a serving is by calculating the amount of product it would take to render less than 5 calories. If, for example, a BBQ flavored seasoning contains 4 calories worth of brown sugar in ¼ of a teaspoon, the **Nutrition Facts Table** would list '**Serving Size ¼ teaspoon** with '**Calories 0**' and '**Sugars 0**'. In this instance, upon reading the ingredient label, one would see 'dextrose' (another name for sugar) as the second ingredient listed in the seasoning's make up. Keep in mind that ingredients are listed in order of percentage of composition. In this particular case, salt was the main ingredient with sugar as the second ingredient.

Second, even if there is some undetected sugar, how could a few granules in steak seasoning or garlic salt inhibit weight loss? Remember that when a person is taking HCG, his/her system is an 'open system', not at all like a person who is not under the influence of HCG. An 'open system' is extremely sensitive to fats, starches, chemicals and sugars and even a miniscule amount can absolutely have a negative effect on weight loss.

What is a person to do? Forget the **Nutrition Fact Table** and read the **Ingredients** to see if fat, starch or sugar is part of the seasoning composition. There should be no type of oil (such as soybean or canola oil), no type of starch (such as corn starch or flour) and no type of sugar.

There are numerous names for sugar. The list below reveals many of them. In spices, the most common are: any type of sugar (ex. Beet sugar, brown sugar), any type of syrup (ex. Corn syrup, Rice syrup), anything ending in 'ose' (ex. Dextrose, fructose), and some ending in 'trin' (ex. Maltodextrin).

Common and Not-so-common names for sugar:

Barbados Sugar	Golden sugar
Barley malt	Golden syrup
Beet sugar	Grape sugar
Brown sugar	High-fructose corn syrup
Buttered syrup	Honey
Cane-juice crystals	Invert sugar
Cane sugar	Lactose
Caramel	Malt
Carob syrup	Malt syrup
Corn syrup	Maltodextrin
Corn syrup solids	Maltose
Date sugar	Mannitol
Demerara Sugar	Molasses
Dextran	Muscovado
Dextrose	Panocha
Diatase	Refiner's syrup
Diastatic malt	Rice Syrup
Ethyl maltol	Sorbitol
Fructose	Sorghum syrup
Fruit juice	Sucrose
Fruit juice concentrate	Sugar
galactose	Treacle
Glucose	Turbinado sugar
Glucose solids	Yellow sugar

Regarding spices, Dr. Simeons states that "The juice of one lemon daily is allowed for all purposes. Salt, pepper, vinegar, mustard powder, garlic, sweet basil, parsley, thyme, marjoram, etc. may be used for seasoning, but no oil, butter or dressing." Our interpretation of his guideline in making use of spices is that the spice is allowable if it is in its pure form, either fresh or dried, either stand alone or combined with other allowable spices.

Additionally, we contend that an item may be classified as a spice or a vegetable depending upon which form it takes. We base the distinction on this determining factor, "Does it dissolve when added to liquid?" If yes, it's a spice, if not, it is a vegetable. We consider dehydrated onions as a vegetable, but onion powder as a spice. Keep in mind also that onion is an allowable vegetable, but never the less, it is still a vegetable and Dr. Simeons stipulates ONLY ONE TYPE OF VEGETABLE. While peppers are NOT on the list of allowable vegetables, ground pepper, per Dr. Simeons, is an allowable spice.

For those people who, for whatever reason, don't want to determine or worry about the 'allowability' of the spices they use for this phase of the diet, they may purchase the following which as of April, 2008 contain no fat, starch or sugar. We have not analyzed all available seasonings on the market but here are a few that you can definitely use.

McCormick Garlic Pepper Grinder
McCormick Italian Seasoning
Reese All Purpose Steak Salt
Spice Island Herbes De Provence
Spice Island Ground Chipotle Chile
Tony Chachere's Original Creole Seasoning

In addition, you can use the following at your discretion. They have no fat, starch or sugar but the label lists one ingredient common to all of these seasonings as 'onion', not stipulating if the onion is extracted, ground, or dehydrated. They do, however, pass the 'dissolve test' so the only point in question is if vegetable types are being mixed.

McCormick Steakhouse Seasoning Grinder
McCormick Italian Herb Seasoning Grinder
McCormick Broiled Steak Seasoning Salt
McCormick Rotisserie Chicken Seasoning
McCormick Herb Chicken Seasoning
Spice Classic Soul Food Seasoning Salt
Spice Classic Steak Seasoning Salt
Spice Classic Poultry Seasoning
Weber Grill Creations N'Orleans Cajun Seasoning

Some frequent violators are garlic salt, paprika, most seasoning mixes (Lawry's, and other well-known), and many other, common spices – you must check ALL spice labels – even the ones that simply state PAPRIKA or one other 'ingredient' on the face of the container.

Be mindful of this information and have a flavorful day!

Beverages

Orange Slushy (Picture K on Cover)

¾ c. crushed ice
1 orange
5 drops Valencia Orange flavored stevia

Mix in blender until smooth. Pour into glass and serve.
Servings: 1 fruit

Orange Julius (Picture K on cover)

¾ c. crushed ice
1 orange
5 drops Valencia Orange flavored stevia
5 drops Vanilla Crème flavored stevia

Mix in blender until smooth. Pour into glass and serve.
Servings: 1 fruit

Strawberry Orange Smoothie

¾ c. crushed ice
1 orange
1 c. fresh or partially defrosted strawberries
5 drops Clear stevia
5 drops Valencia Orange stevia
5 drops Vanilla Crème stevia

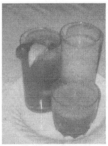

Picture K on Cover

Mix in blender until smooth. Pour into glass and serve or freeze to
make shaved ice.
Servings: 2 fruits

Lemonade

1 c. water   5 drops Clear stevia
1 T. fresh lemon juice   15 drops Lemon stevia

Stir in glass and add ice to serve or freeze to make shaved ice.
Servings: 0 fruit (Allowed the juice from 1 fresh lemon per day.)

Strawberry Lemonade

½ c. crushed ice
1 c. water
1 T. fresh lemon juice
7 to10 small-medium fresh or partially defrosted strawberries
25 drops Lemon flavored stevia
10 drops Clear stevia

Mix in blender until smooth. Pour into glass and serve or freeze to make shaved ice.
Servings: 1 fruit

Iced Raspberry Coffee

1 ½ c. crushed ice
½ c. strong coffee
5 drops Chocolate Raspberry stevia
1 T. milk
10 drops Vanilla Crème stevia

Mix in blender until smooth. Pour into glass and serve.
Servings: 1 milk

Frozen Cappuccino

1 c. crushed ice
1 T. milk
5 drops Vanilla Crème stevia
5 drops English Toffee stevia
5 drops Clear stevia

Mix in blender until smooth. Pour into glass and serve.
Servings: 1 milk

Hot Chocolate

8 oz. hot water
5 drops Chocolate stevia
2 drops Vanilla Crème stevia

Hot Raspberry Chocolate

8 oz. hot water
4 drops Chocolate Raspberry stevia
3 drops Vanilla Crème stevia

Cinnamon Dolce

1 c. crushed ice
1 T. milk
5 drops Vanilla Crème stevia
5 drops English Toffee stevia
5 drops Clear stevia
5 drops Cinnamon stevia
Mix in blender until smooth.
Pour into glass and serve.
Servings: 1 milk

Soda

The soda recipes are made with carbonated water as the base. We used the Mendota sparkling water brand but any plain non sweetened carbonated water will do. The sweetener/flavoring we used is SWEET LEAF brand flavored stevia. Please refer to the article on stevia in this book (pg. 4).

Keep in mind that stevia is one of those things that people tend to either love or hate. Therefore, people think that these soft drinks either taste exactly like the originals or ... they don't!

Root Beer

8 oz. carbonated water
15 drops Root Beer stevia

Root Beer Crème

8 oz. carbonated water
13 drops Root Beer stevia
3 drops Vanilla Crème stevia

Orange Soda

8 oz. carbonated water
15 drops Valencia Orange stevia

Mock Fresca

8 oz. carbonated water
10 drops Lemon Drop stevia

Citrus Burst

8 oz. carbonated water
10 drops Lemon Drop stevia
5 drops Apricot Nectar stevia

Grape

8 oz. carbonated water
10 drops Grape stevia

Mock 7-UP

8 oz. carbonated water
10 drops Valencia Orange stevia

Flavored Water

If you do not like the taste of the sparkling mineral water, but like flavored water, any of the above recipes can be used with plain/ bottled water. The amount of stevia required for flavor would be less, so experiment and enjoy.

Fruits

Apple Cobbler

1 sliced apple
1/8 t. cinnamon
1 packet stevia
Toss the above ingredients and arrange
on a microwave safe plate.

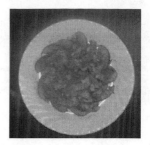

Picture W on back cover

Topping:
2 Classic flavored Melba Toast rounds
Cinnamon
¼ packet stevia

Sprinkle apples with crumbled Melba Toast rounds, cinnamon and
¼ packet stevia. Heat in microwave on high for 2 minutes.
Servings: 1 fruit, 1 starch

Fruit Medley (Picture O on cover – side dish)

1 orange
7 to10 small-medium strawberries
1 packet stevia (optional depending upon the sweetness of the fruit)

Toss cut up orange and sliced strawberries. Sprinkle stevia to taste.
Servings: 2 fruits

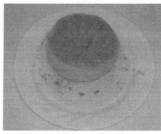

Jamaican Grapefruit

½ grapefruit
Cinnamon
1-2 packets stevia

Picture AA on back cover

Using a serrated edge knife, cut grapefruit in half as normally would
and place on a microwave safe plate. Cut around center core, rind,
and partitions. Sprinkle with cinnamon and stevia. Heat in
microwave on high for 2 minutes.
Servings: 1 fruit

Apples with Strawberry Sauce

½ Jonathon apple
3 to 5 small-medium strawberries
3 drops Vanilla Crème stevia

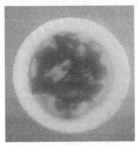

Picture R on back cover

Slice apple and arrange on a plate. Mash the strawberries with a fork and add Vanilla Crème stevia to make a sauce. Pour over the apple slices.
Servings: 1 fruit

Homemade Applesauce

5 apples (Jonathon, Gala, Fuji)
1 t. fresh lemon juice
½ c. water
1 packet stevia
½ t. cinnamon

Peel, core and chop apples. Cook apples and water in a crock pot on low for 2 hours. When cooled, puree apples in blender while adding stevia and cinnamon. Divide into 5 equal portions (usually about ½ c. per serving).
Servings: 5 fruits

Strawberries and Crème

7 to 10 small-medium strawberries
1 T. milk
1 drop Vanilla Crème stevia
1 packet stevia

Slice strawberries and toss with packet of stevia to taste. Measure milk into separate bowl and stir in liquid stevia. Pour over strawberries.
Servings: 1 fruit, 1 milk

Salad Dressings

Vinaigrette Dressing

¼ c. apple cider vinegar
½ c. water
2 shakes celery salt
2 shakes onion salt
Ground pepper to taste
20 drops Clear stevia
3 packets stevia

Combine ingredients, pour into jar and refrigerate.

Lemon Dressing

¼ c. apple cider vinegar
1 c. water
1 T. fresh lemon juice
25 drops Clear stevia
1 packet of stevia

Combine ingredients, pour into jar and refrigerate.

Citrus Dressing

¼ c. apple cider vinegar
1 c. water
1 T. fresh lemon juice
15 drops Clear stevia
10 drops Apricot Nectar flavored stevia
1 packet of stevia
¼ t. Chinese Style Five Spice (Optional)
¼ t. garlic salt (Optional)

Combine ingredients, pour into jar and refrigerate.

Seasoning Mixes

Cajun Dry Rub Seasoning

8 T. paprika
3 T. cayenne
6 T. ground black pepper
4 T. garlic granules** (or 2 T. garlic powder)
3 T. onion granules** (or 1-1/2 T. onion powder)
6 T. sea salt
2 T. ground cumin
4 T. dried oregano
4 T. dried thyme

Combine all the ingredients, blending well. Store in an airtight container away from heat and light. Dry rub seasonings can be rubbed into meat, fish, or poultry or added to gumbos, pastas, or almost any dish that you want to spice up. Perfect as a seasoning for fried or grilled chicken, chicken pasta dishes or gumbo.
Makes about 2-1/2 cups

Classic Poultry Seasoning

1 T. onion powder
1 T. garlic powder
2 T. dried sage leaves, crumbled or whole
2 T. dried thyme leaves
2 T. dried parsley leaves

Combine all of the ingredients in a bowl and blend. Put in container with a tight fitting lid and store away from heat and light. Shake or stir to re-blend before each use.

This tangy blend of herbs is just right for roast chicken, fried chicken, or most any chicken or poultry dish where you want flavor – not heat.
Makes 2/3 cup

Cajun Poultry Seasoning

2 T. paprika
¾ T. cayenne
1 ½ T. ground black pepper
3 T. garlic granules
1 ½ T. onion powder
1 ½ T. sea salt
½ T. ground cumin
1 T. dried oregano
3 T. dried thyme leaves
2 T. dried sage leaves, crumbled or whole
2 T. dried parsley leaves

For a finer texture, pour all ingredients in a food processor and
pulse several times. Store seasoning blends in an airtight
container, away from heat and light. For best flavor, use within
3 – 4 months.
Makes 1 ¼ cup

All Purpose Seasoning

1 T. sea salt
1 T. garlic powder
1 T. onion powder
½ T. black pepper

Combine in a small bowl and store in an airtight container, away
from heat and light.

Southwest Seasoning

1 T. chili powder   ½ t. paprika
¼ t. garlic powder   1½ t. ground cumin
¼ t. onion powder   1 t. sea salt
¼ t. dried oregano   1 t. black pepper

In a small bowl, mix together chili powder, garlic powder, onion
powder, oregano, paprika, cumin, salt and pepper. Store in an air
tight container away from heat and light.

Salads

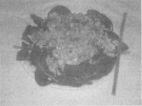

Tasty Chicken Apple Salad

2 c. raw spinach or romaine lettuce
½ c. chopped apple
100 grams chicken breast
Vinaigrette, Lemon or Citrus Dressing (pg. 13)

Picture H on cover

Cook and chop chicken. Arrange spinach or lettuce on plate, sprinkle with chopped apple and chopped chicken. Spray or spoon on Vinaigrette, Lemon or Citrus Dressing.
Servings: 1 protein, 1 vegetable, ½ fruit

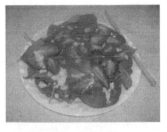

Strawberry Chicken Salad

2 c. raw spinach or romaine lettuce
3 to 5 small-medium sliced strawberries
100 grams chicken breast
Vinaigrette Dressing (pg. 13)

Picture U on back cover

Cook and chop chicken. Arrange spinach or lettuce on plate, sprinkle with chopped chicken and strawberries. Spray or spoon on Vinaigrette Dressing.
Servings: 1 protein, 1 vegetable, ½ fruit

Asian Salad

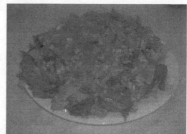

Picture A on cover

2 c. romaine lettuce
½ chopped orange
100 grams chicken breast
¼ t. Chinese Five Spice
1/8 t. garlic salt
1 packet stevia
2 Sesame flavored Melba Toast rounds
Citrus Dressing (pg. 13)

Cook and chop chicken. Toss lettuce, orange, and chicken with
Chinese Five Spice, garlic salt, and stevia. Sprinkle with
crumbled sesame rounds. Spray or spoon on Citrus Dressing.
Servings: 1 protein, 1 vegetable, ½ fruit

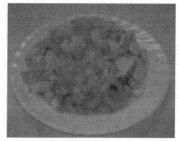

Crunchy Chicken Salad

100 grams chicken breast
½ chopped apple
1 or 2 stalks chopped celery

Picture F on cover

Vinaigrette, Lemon or Citrus Dressing (pg. 13)

Cook and chunk chicken. Toss chicken, apple and celery. Spray
or spoon on Vinaigrette, Lemon or Citrus Dressing.
Servings: 1 protein, 1 vegetable, ½ fruit

Spicy Taco Salad

2 c. romaine lettuce
100 grams 93% fat free ground beef
¼ t. garlic salt
¼ t. chili seasoning
2 Onion flavored Melba Toast rounds
Vinaigrette Dressing (pg. 13)

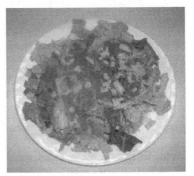

Picture BB on back cover

Prepare ground beef on George Foreman grill. Crumble beef and mix in garlic salt and chili seasoning. Top lettuce with ground beef mixture. Spray or spoon on Vinaigrette Dressing and sprinkle with crumbled Melba rounds.
Servings: 1 protein, 1 vegetable

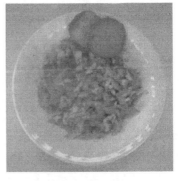

Delightful Crab Salad

100 grams crab meat*
(7 oz. of crab legs including the shells)
 *Do **not** use imitation crab meat.
1 stalk coarsely chopped celery
2 T. Vinaigrette dressing (pg. 13)

Picture X on back cover

Steam crab legs for about 4 minutes. Remove crab meat from shells and chop. Toss with celery and dressing.
Servings: 1 protein, 1 vegetable

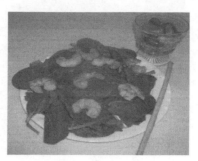

Picture O on cover

Shrimp-Spinach Salad

2 c. raw spinach or romaine lettuce
100 grams grilled shrimp
Dash of garlic salt
Vinaigrette Dressing (pg. 13)

Grill shrimp with dash of garlic salt. Arrange spinach on plate and add shrimp. Spray or spoon on Vinaigrette Dressing.
Servings: 1 protein, 1 vegetable

Soups

Chicken Bouillon Base
(This is used in many recipes in this book.)

6 100 gram pieces of chicken breast
8 c. water
¼ t. garlic powder
¼ t. onion salt
¼ t. celery salt
¼ t. poultry seasoning
¼ t. black pepper
1 ½ t. sea salt

Combine ingredients in soup pot and cook until chicken is done.
Remove chicken and refrigerate or freeze to use at a later time (6
servings). Also freeze bouillon base for future cooking. Put 2
cups in a medium size container to make soups or 4 tablespoons
in a small container to sauté vegetables.

Grandma Simeons' Chicken Soup

2 c. Chicken Bouillon Base (above)
3 stalks coarsely chopped celery
100 grams chopped cooked chicken breast

Cook combined ingredients on medium until celery is tender.
Servings: 1 protein, 1 vegetable

French Onion Soup – Delicious!

2 c. Chicken Bouillon Base (above)
1 whole sliced sweet onion

Simmer on low for 1 hour.
Servings: 1 vegetable

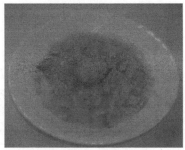

Picture T on back cover

20

Tangy Tomato Soup

1 c. Chicken Bouillon Base (pg. 20)	
1 large or 2 small tomatoes	½ - 1 packet stevia
1 clove minced garlic	½ t. basil
½ t. onion salt	Ground pepper

Sautee garlic in 1 T. of bouillon base and set aside. Puree tomatoes in blender and then cook over medium heat to a boil, stirring frequently. Turn heat to low. Add remaining bouillon base, garlic, onion salt and stevia to tomatoes. Cover and simmer for 10 minutes. Stir in basil, pour in soup bowl and sprinkle with ground pepper to serve.
Servings: 1 vegetable

Beef Onion Bouillon

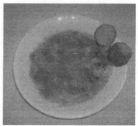

Picture I on cover

2 c. Chicken Bouillon Base (pg. 20)
1 whole sliced sweet onion
100 grams 93% fat free ground beef

Prepare ground beef on George Foreman grill.
Simmer combined ingredients on low for 1 hour.
Servings: 1 protein, 1 vegetable

Chicken Asparagus Soup

100 grams chicken breast
2 c. Chicken Bouillon Base (pg. 20)
8 oz. fresh asparagus
2 t. fresh ginger
½ t. onion salt
½ apple thinly sliced (Optional)

In a large saucepan, combine Chicken Bouillon Base, asparagus, ginger and onion salt. Bring to a boil, then reduce heat. Cover and simmer until asparagus is tender-crisp, about 10 minutes. Add chicken and heat through. To serve, float apple slices on top.
Servings: 1 protein, 1 vegetable, ½ fruit (Optional)

Chicken or Beef Cabbage Soup

2 c. Chicken Bouillon Base (pg. 20)
100 grams chunked cooked chicken breast OR beef
2 c. chopped cabbage
1/8 t. sea salt

Cook combined ingredients on medium until cabbage is tender.
Servings: 1 protein, 1 vegetable

Tomato Beef Soup

100 grams 93% fat free ground beef
1 large or 2 small tomatoes
1 clove garlic
1 ½ packets stevia
1/8 t. onion salt
Sea salt to taste

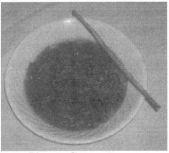

Picture G on cover

Combine chopped tomato, minced garlic, spices and crumbled
ground beef prepared on a George Foreman grill. Sautee until
heated through.
Servings: 1 protein, 1 vegetable

Fish Soup with Garlic

100 grams of cod cut into 1 inch cubes
1 minced clove garlic
½ t. oregano
½ t. thyme
1 large or 2 small tomatoes
2 c. Chicken Bouillon Base (pg. 20)
Sea salt
Pepper

Sautee garlic in 2 T. of the bouillon base. Add the rest of the
bouillon and chopped tomatoes. After coming to a boil, reduce
heat to simmer. Add fresh herbs and salt and pepper to taste.
Add fish cubes and cook for 5-7 minutes or until fish is cooked.
Servings: 1 protein, 1 vegetable

Vegetables

Cucumber Salad

1 large cucumber
4 T. apple cider vinegar
¼ t. garlic powder
1/8 t. pepper

½ t. onion salt
1 T. dried parsley
1 packet stevia

Combine vinegar with spices and stevia. Toss cucumbers with vinegar mixture and refrigerate for at least 1 hour.
Servings: 1 vegetable

Cream Spinach

4 T. Chicken Bouillon Base (pg. 20)
2 drops Vanilla Crème flavored stevia
3 c. raw spinach

Heat bouillon base and stevia on medium to just prior to boiling. Add spinach and sauté a few minutes until tender.
Servings: 1 vegetable

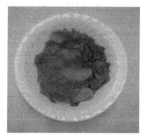

Red Chard, Apple and Cinnamon   Picture CC on back cover

6 T. water
¼ t. cinnamon
Pinch of nutmeg
Pinch of allspice
Pinch of salt

Pinch of pepper
4 drops Cinnamon stevia
2 c. chopped red chard leaves
½ apple sliced thin

Add spices to heated water. Fold the chard and apples gently into the mixture and cook over medium heat for about 5 minutes.
Servings: 1 vegetable, ½ fruit

Creole Cucumbers

2 c. sliced cucumbers
1/8 t. Creole Seasoning

Mix and serve.
Servings: 1 vegetable

Lemon Garlic Chard

2 c. roughly chopped Swiss chard
1 large or 2 small sliced garlic cloves
4 T. water
Fresh lemon juice
Sea salt
Pepper

Put 1 T. water in non stick pan. Sautee garlic until tender and set aside. Pour remaining water into pan and add chard. Cook over medium heat for about 5 minutes, tossing occasionally. Drain off excess juice and return to pan adding in sautéed garlic. Before serving, give a squirt of lemon juice and a shake of salt and pepper.
Servings: 1 vegetable

Minted Cucumbers

1 large cucumber   Onion salt
1 minced garlic clove   Pepper
2 T. fresh lemon juice
2 T. chopped fresh mint or ½ t. crushed dried mint leaves

Cut cucumbers in half lengthwise, remove seeds and dice. Mix cucumber with garlic, lemon juice and mint. Season with onion salt and pepper. Refrigerate for 45 minutes.
Toss before serving and garnish with whole fresh mint leaves.
Servings: 1 vegetable

Cucumber Apple Salad

½ chopped apple
1 sliced cucumber
2 T. apple cider vinegar
1 T. water

Garlic salt
Pepper
Stevia (Optional)

Chop apple and thinly slice cucumber. Combine vinegar and water. Season with garlic salt, pepper and stevia (optional) to taste.
Servings: 1 vegetable, ½ fruit

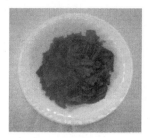

Beet Greens

4 T. Chicken Bouillon Base (pg. 20)
2 c. chopped beet greens
Dash of onion salt

Picture N on cover

Heat bouillon base on medium to just prior to boiling. Reduce heat, add greens and sauté a few minutes until tender. Sprinkle with onion salt.
Servings: 1 vegetable

Grilled Onions

1 whole sweet onion   Sea salt

Slice sweet onion and place on preheated George Foreman grill. Sprinkle with sea salt. Grill 4-5 minutes until onions are tender and juicy. Note: Grilling onions with any meat will deliciously flavor both the onions and the meat.
Servings: 1 vegetable

Lemon Zest Asparagus

1/3 lb. asparagus   Sea salt
1 T. fresh lemon juice   Ground pepper

Prepare the asparagus by rinsing thoroughly and breaking off any tough, white bottoms. Cut into 1 to 2 inch sections, slicing the asparagus at a slight diagonal.
Fill a medium sized saucepan half way with water and bring to a boil. Add the asparagus and reduce heat slightly to a simmer. Parboil the asparagus for exactly 2 minutes. Drain the hot water. While the asparagus are still hot, toss them in a bowl with lemon juice. Salt and pepper to taste. Serve warm or room temperature.
Servings: 1 vegetable

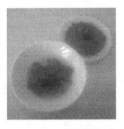

Citrus Tomato Salsa   **Picture DD on back cover**

1 large or 2 small tomatoes   3 drops Clear stevia
1 T. fresh lemon juice   1 t. chopped fresh cilantro
1/8 t. celery salt   1/8 t. garlic powder
1/8 t. chili powder   1/8 c. Vinaigrette dressing (pg. 13)

Chop tomatoes. Combine dressing, lemon juice, spices and stevia. Toss in tomato and refrigerate for at least 1 hour.
Servings: 1 vegetable

Slaw

2 c. shredded cabbage or lettuce
Vinaigrette dressing (pg. 13)
Toss cabbage with dressing. Chill for 10 minutes.
Servings: 1 vegetable

Radish Salad

2 T. fresh lemon juice
3 drops Clear stevia
1 ½ c. thinly sliced radishes
½ thinly sliced apple

1 T. chopped fresh dill
Sea salt
Pepper

Combine stevia and lemon juice in a bowl. Add radish and apple.
Toss slices in juice mixture and season with dill, salt and pepper.
Servings: 1 vegetable, ½ fruit

Sautéed Baby Spinach

½ bag baby spinach
1 clove minced garlic
4 T. Chicken Bouillon Base (pg. 20) or water

Make sure to use baby spinach since regular spinach will be a
little bitter. Sauté garlic in 1 T. of the Chicken Bouillon Base or
water.

Add remaining bouillon base or water and spinach, and toss until
covered in garlic mixture and starts to get soft. Remove before it
cooks down to mush.
Servings: 1 vegetable

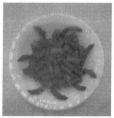

Picture V on back cover

Asparagus Salad

2 c. asparagus
Vinaigrette dressing (pg. 13)
100 grams cooked chicken or seafood (Optional)

Steam asparagus, cool, then cut in 1 inch pieces.
Toss in Vinaigrette dressing and chill. For a complete meal, add
chicken or seafood.
Servings: 1vegetable, 1 protein (Optional)

Baked Vidalia Onion

1 Vidalia onion (or any sweet onion)
Sea Salt
Pepper

Remove the outer layers and roots from the onion. Wrap the onion in foil. Bake in a preheated oven at 350 for at least 1 hour (medium size onion). Remove from foil and season with salt and pepper.
Servings: 1 vegetable

Entrees

Beef Entrees

Choosing cuts of Beef – The best cuts of steak for this phase of the HCG diet are: filet mignon, flank steak, T-bone, top round, top sirloin and tenderloin with all visible fat removed.

The best cuts of roast for this phase of the HCG diet are: bottom round, eye of round, and sirloin tip.

If you are going to eat ground beef, it should be, at a minimum, 93% fat free and eaten no more than 2 or 3 times a week.

Veal with Grilled Onions

1 whole sliced sweet onion
100 grams veal

Acquire veal from a chop, removing all visible fat. Do not use ground veal as the fat content is too high. Sandwich meat between onions on George Foreman grill. Sprinkle meat and onions with sea salt.

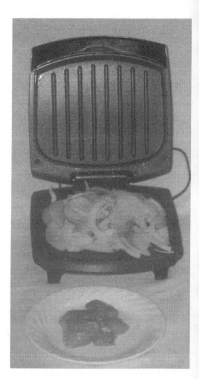

Works equally well with veal, beef, and chicken.

Servings: 1 protein, 1 vegetable

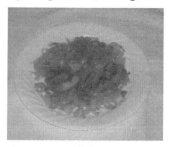

Picture B on cover

Bunless Burgers

100 grams 93% fat free ground beef
1 large tomato
Onion salt
Ground pepper
Dill seed

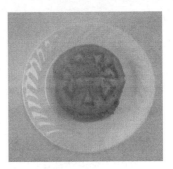

Prepare ground beef patty on George Foreman grill. Cut
horizontally so have 2 thin patties. Sandwich each patty between
2 slices of tomato. Sprinkle with onion salt, ground pepper and a
tiny bit of dill seed. Serve with sliced tomatoes for the rest of
your vegetable.
Servings: 1 protein, 1 vegetable

Garlic Italian Roast

3 lb lean beef roast, fat removed
6-8 large cloves garlic
1 t. dry oregano
1 t. sea salt
Fresh ground pepper
Water
1/6 head of cabbage OR 1 sweet onion (Optional)

Cooking for the gang? Place the above in roaster, add water until
it is about 1½ inches deep, and bake for 15 min. on 350.
Optionally, add potatoes and carrots for 'the gang' and cabbage
OR a sweet onion for the HCG Dieter. Continue baking an
additional 45-60 minutes depending upon how done you like
your roast. Slice off 3 oz. of lean roast with all visible fat
removed for the HCG dieter.
Servings: 3 oz. cooked = 1 protein, 1 vegetable (Optional)

Italian Beef

100 grams 93% fat free ground beef
1 large or 2 small tomatoes chopped
1 minced clove garlic
¼ t. garlic salt
¼ t. Italian seasoning
1 packet stevia

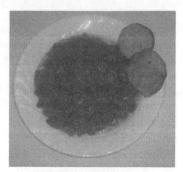

Picture L on cover

Prepare ground beef on George Foreman grill. Sauté garlic in a little juice from the tomato. Toss crumbled beef with other ingredients and add to sauté pan. Remove from stove when heated, before tomatoes cook down too much.
Servings: 1 protein, 1 vegetable

Beef Curry

100 grams very lean steak cut into 1 in. cubes

1 whole sliced sweet onion	1 shake turmeric
½ clove minced garlic	2 shakes pepper
½ t. minced fresh ginger	4 shakes sea salt
¼ t. ground coriander	4 T. water
1/8 t. ground cumin	2 t. chopped cilantro

In a large frying pan, heat 3 T. water over moderate heat. Add the onion and cook, stirring occasionally, until translucent, about 5 minutes. Add the garlic and ginger and cook, stirring, for 1 minute. Meanwhile, in a small bowl, combine the coriander, cumin, turmeric, pepper, salt, and 1 T. water. Add the paste to the onion and cook, stirring, for 1 minute.

Add the meat to the pan and cook, stirring, for 3 minutes. Raise the heat to moderately high and cook to your taste, stirring, about 2 minutes longer for medium rare. Stir in the cilantro.

Note: A long-simmering curry becomes a quick one when you substitute a tender cut of beef (sirloin, fillet...) and stir-fry it till medium-rare.
Servings: 1 protein, 1 vegetable

Beef Lettuce Cups

100 grams lean steak
1 T. water
1 shake ginger
½ clove crushed garlic

1 pinch Chinese Five Spice
1 shake chili seasoning
2 crisp lettuce cups

Cut steak into thin slivers and put in a bowl. Add water, ginger, garlic, five-spice powder and chili seasoning. Mix well, then cover and marinate in refrigerator for 1 hour, stirring occasionally Add beef mixture to non stick pan and stir-fry for 2-3 minutes, stirring all the time. Turn mixture into a warm serving dish. Serve at once by simply spooning beef mixture into lettuce cups and eat with fingers. Serve with plenty of napkins or finger bowls - it can be a little messy.
Servings: 1 protein, 1 vegetable

Spicy Beef Kabobs

100 grams lean beef sirloin
½ clove chopped garlic
1/8 t. paprika
2 shakes cayenne pepper
1/8 t. cumin (roasted)
1/8 tsp. coarse salt
1/8 t. ground pepper
1 T. apple cider vinegar
12-inch metal skewers
1 sweet onion OR 1 large tomato (Optional)

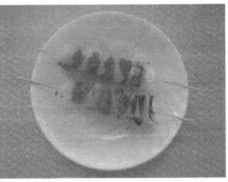

Picture S on back cover

Cut beef into 1½-inch cubes. Combine spices and vinegar. Place meat in a sealable plastic bag with the marinade; squeeze excess air from bag. Place bag in refrigerator for 4 hours, turning once or twice. After 4 hours, remove meat and place on metal skewers, leaving a little space in between. Grill on medium heat about 12 minutes (allow 3 minutes for each of the four sides.) Remove to aluminum foil and wrap. Allow to cool 3-4 minutes before serving. For a complete meal, add chunks of sweet onion to the kabob and on the side.
Servings: 1 protein, 1 vegetable (Optional)

Veal Chops

1 c. Chicken Bouillon Base (pg. 20)
½ clove minced garlic
½ t. dried crushed oregano leaves
3 100 gram veal chop pieces
1/4 c. cold Chicken Bouillon Base (pg. 20)

Cut veal pieces from the chop, removing all visible fat. Do not use ground veal as the fat content is too high. Combine Chicken Bouillon Base, garlic, and oregano. Place veal pieces in a shallow bowl or heavy plastic bag. Pour mixture over veal pieces. Refrigerate for 2 to 4 hours, turning occasionally.

Drain veal; reserve marinade. In skillet over medium heat, brown veal pieces in a small amount of the reserved marinade. Reduce heat; cover and simmer for 30 minutes, or until tender.
Servings: 3 proteins

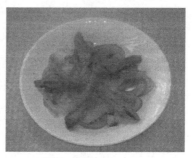

Peppercorn Steak   Picture D on cover

4 100 gram lean beef steak pieces
30 whole peppercorns, cracked
1/3 t. salt
2 T. water
1 large or 2 medium sweet onions

Crack pepper by placing in a towel and striking it with a wooden mallet or rolling pin. Moisten steaks and then pat cracked pepper and salt onto steaks. Heat water in a nonstick pan. Place steaks and sliced onion in the pan and brown 15 minutes.
Servings: 4 proteins

Chicken Entrees

Mock Egg Roll

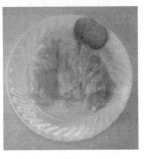

2-3 big cabbage leaves
1 c. shredded cabbage
1/8 t. onion salt
1/8 t. garlic powder
1/8 t. Chinese Five Spice
½ packet stevia
2 Sesame flavored Melba Toast rounds
100 grams cooked chopped chicken or shrimp

Picture E on cover

Steam big cabbage leaves for 5 minutes. Move leaves over to side of steamer to make room for shredded cabbage. Steam both for 5 minutes. Remove shredded cabbage to a mixing bowl. Add chopped chicken or shrimp and spices. Mix and then wrap in big cabbage leaves. Garnish with Melba rounds.

As this recipe calls for only 1 cup of cabbage, feel free to have an additional cup of shredded cabbage uncooked with the vinaigrette dressing (slaw).
Servings: 1 protein, ½ vegetable

Cajun Chicken

4 100 gram pieces of chicken breast
1 T. Cajun Poultry Seasoning (pg. 15)
1/8 t. pepper
¼ t. salt
¼ t. onion powder
¼ t. garlic powder
½ T. water

Combine the seasonings and water to form a paste, adding more water if needed. Rub all over the chicken pieces; place in a zip lock bag and refrigerate for at least 1 hour. Grill or broil the chicken for about 5 to 7 minutes on each side, depending on thickness. Chicken is done when juices run clear when pricked with a fork.
Servings: 4 proteins

Chicken Fajitas

2 T. apple cider vinegar
1 t. minced garlic
1 T. fresh lemon juice
1 t. cumin
1 t. pepper
1 t. sea salt
½ t. onion salt
½ t. celery salt
¼ t. chili powder
3 drops Clear stevia
2 100 gram chicken breast pieces

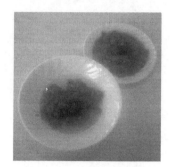

Picture DD on back cover

Slice raw chicken into strips. Mix ingredients for marinade and place in a sealable bag with chicken strips. Refrigerate for about 8 hours, turning occasionally. Pan fry chicken in a nonstick pan. Arrange chicken strips on plate and top with Citrus Tomato Salsa (p. 26) (Optional).
Servings: 1 protein, 1 vegetable (Optional)

Italian Chicken Kabobs

100 grams chicken breast
¼ c. Vinaigrette Dressing (pg. 13)
1 t. Italian Seasoning
1 sweet onion

Cut chicken into 1 ½ inch cubes. Cut onion into small wedges. Combine dressing and seasoning and place in a sealable bag with the meat and onion wedges. Place bag in refrigerator for 4 hours, turning once or twice. After 4 hours, remove meat and onion and place on metal skewers leaving a little space in between. Grill on medium heat.
Servings: 1 protein, 1 vegetable

Fried Chicken

100 grams chicken breast Sea salt
1 T. milk Pepper
1 Grissini breadstick

Totally crush breadstick in food processor or put in a plastic bag
and crush with a rolling pin. Dip chicken in milk and coat with
breadstick crumbs. Cook in a nonstick pan.
Season with salt and pepper.
Servings: 1 protein

Blackened Chicken

100 grams chicken breast 1/8 t. onion powder
1/8 t. salt 1/4 t. ground cumin
1/8 t. garlic powder 1/8 t. cayenne pepper
1/8 t. ground black pepper 1/8 t. paprika
1/8 t. white pepper

Pound chicken breast to about 1/3" thick. Combine seasoning
mix ingredients in a small bowl. Just before cooking piece of
chicken, moisten with water and sprinkle the fillet evenly with
the seasoning mix, patting it in with your hands. Immediately
place the fillet flat in a hot non stick skillet. If you are making
more than one serving, place each fillet in the skillet before
seasoning another one.

Cook uncovered over the same high heat until the underside
forms a crust, about 2 minutes. (The time will vary according to
the thickness of the fillet and the heat of the skillet or fire; watch
the meat and you'll see a white line coming up the side as it
cooks.) Turn the fillet over. Cook just until meat is cooked
through, about 2 more minutes. Serve the chicken fillet crustier
side up while piping hot.
Servings: 1 protein

Baked Garlic Chicken

4 100 gram pieces of chicken breast
3 t. crushed garlic cloves
2 T. water   ½ t. oregano
Dash of salt   ½ t. basil
Dash of pepper

Put the garlic and water into the microwave for 20 seconds. Add
salt, pepper and herbs to form a paste, adding more water if
needed. Rub all over the chicken pieces. Lay the chicken pieces
in a baking pan and bake on 425 for 30 minutes.
Servings: 4 proteins

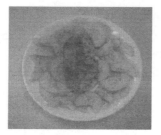

Picture Z on back cover

Lemon Chicken with Roasted Garlic

4 100 gram pieces of chicken breast washed and patted dry
¼ c. Chicken Bouillon Base (pg. 20)
3 T. fresh lemon juice   1½ t. dried oregano
2 T. water   Sea salt
5-7 whole peeled garlic cloves   Pepper

Preheat oven to 400 degrees. Place the garlic in a roasting pan.
Lay the chicken pieces over the garlic cloves. Top the chicken
with the remaining ingredients and season well with salt and
pepper. Roast in 400 degree oven, turning occasionally until the
chicken is golden and most of the broth/juice has evaporated.
Remove the chicken from the pan and serve garnished with the
whole roasted garlic cloves and additional lemon wedges.
Servings: 4 proteins

Spicy Baked Chicken

4 100 gram pieces of chicken breast
1 onion
2 cloves garlic
Tony Chachere's Original Creole Seasoning

Season chicken and place in baking pan. Cut onion as desired and place in baking pan. Mince garlic and add to baking pan. Cover with aluminum foil. Bake 35 minutes at 375 or until done.
Servings: 4 proteins, 1 vegetable (if eat the onion)

Grill-a-Batch of Chicken

6 100 gram pieces of chicken breast
Southwest Seasoning (pg. 15)
Classic Poultry Seasoning (pg. 14)
Cajun Poultry Seasoning (pg. 15)

If you're pressed for time, yet appreciate variety, here's a good way to get stocked up for the week. Make three versions of grilled chicken and freeze in snack size baggies.

Moisten chicken pieces. Sprinkle the top of two of them with the Southwest Seasoning, two of them with the Classic Poultry Seasoning and two of them with the Cajun Poultry Seasoning. Fire up your grill to the maximum level and heat it up. Put the chicken pieces on the front of the grill, spice-side down. Turn the front 2 burners off and leave only the back burners on at a low heat. This does a slow cook to the chicken.

Spice the top side of the breasts and let them cook for 30 min. to an hour, checking occasionally. They will be REALLY juicy and flavorful.
Servings: 6 proteins

Shake and Bake Chicken

4 100 gram pieces of chicken breast
¼ t. cracked black pepper   ¼ t. rosemary
¼ t. sea salt   1 packet stevia
¼ t. thyme   1 seasoning bag

Combine all dry spices inside seasoning bag and shake well. Add
chicken pieces, one at a time, and shake well until breasts are
well seasoned. Place chicken on George Foreman grill cooking
on both sides until well browned and done.
Servings: 4 proteins

Chinese Chicken

100 grams chicken cut in ¾ in. cubes (shrimp or a lean steak
would work as well)
5 T. Chicken Bouillon Base (pg. 20)
Cabbage   ½ packet stevia
1 minced clove garlic   Pepper
1/8 t. onion salt   Sea Salt
1/8 t. Chinese Five Spice

Shred cabbage or slice it very thin. Sautee minced garlic in 1 T.
of bouillon base. Add 2 T. of bouillon base and cabbage and stir
fry over medium heat. Remove while still crunchy. Combine 2
T. of bouillon base, onion salt, Chinese Five Spice, and stevia.
Pour into pan with cubed chicken. Stir fry chicken. Throw
cabbage back in for 1-2 minutes until heated. Slide onto serving
dish.
Servings: 1 protein, 1 vegetable

Fish & Seafood Entrees

Allowable Fish - Raw, not pickled or dried - bass, (sea or striped), burbot, cisco, cod Atlantic cod, Pacific cod, cusk, dolphin*, flounder, grouper, haddock, ling, ling cod, mahi-mahi*, monkfish, northern pike, ocean perch (Atlantic), orange roughy, pike, pollock (Atlantic), rockfish (Pacific), rainbow smelt, snapper, sole, tarpon*, tilapia, walleye, whiting, wolfish (Atlantic)

Allowable Seafood – Lobster, shrimp, scallops*, crab (imitation crabmeat is **not** allowed due to sugar content)

* These items meet the nutritional criteria of other 500 calorie phase fish/seafood and are not specifically excluded by Dr. Simeons, but some might consider these questionable. If you want to be conservative, you may wish to avoid these for this phase.

Quick and Easy Lobster & Asparagus

100 grams lobster (about a 5 oz. tail including the shell)
2 c. asparagus
Garlic salt
Sea salt

Put lobster tail in steamer with asparagus. Sprinkle with garlic salt and sea salt.
Servings: 1 protein, 1 vegetable

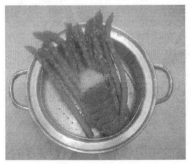

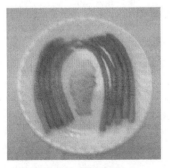

Before   **After – Picture M on cover**

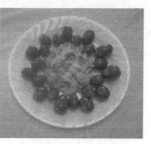

Picture C on cover

Steamed Crab Legs

100 grams crab
(about 7 oz. of crab legs including the shells)
Steam about 4 minutes. Remove from shells.

Optional: Shown with grape tomatoes (1 vegetable)
Servings: 1 protein

Fish in a Bag

4 Sheets of parchment paper
2 100 gram pieces of allowable fish (ex. Tilapia)
4 c. fresh Spinach, washed and dried
4 T. Vinaigrette, Lemon or Citrus Dressing (pg. 13)
All-Purpose Seasoning (pg. 15)

Cooking fish in a parchment bag results in a moist, flaky fish.
Place 2 c. spinach in the center of each of 2 of the parchment
paper pieces. Top each spinach stack with 1 T. dressing. Place
one piece of fish on top of the spinach mixture. Sprinkle with
seasoning and top with 1 T. dressing. Place one sheet of the
parchment on top of each piece of the fish. Crimp the two sheets
of parchment paper like a piecrust until the bottom and the top
are completely sealed.

Place the bags of tilapia onto a cookie sheet and cook in a
preheated 400 degree oven for 15-20 minutes. Place the bag onto
a plate and slice the parchment open at the table to enjoy.
Servings: 2 proteins, 2 vegetables

Simply Broiled Scallops

100 grams scallops
Garlic salt
Fresh lemon juice

Rinse scallops and place in a shallow baking pan. Sprinkle with garlic salt and lemon juice. Broil on medium 6 to 8 minutes. Do not overcook.
Servings: 1 protein

Chilean Sea Bass

4 100 gram Chilean sea bass fillets (or other firm whitefish)
2 cloves garlic, minced ½ lemon
2 T. finely chopped cilantro Salt, pepper, paprika

Arrange Sea bass fillets in a single layer on foil-lined broiler pan. Spread garlic and cilantro on and around fish. Squeeze lemon juice on fillets, sprinkle salt and pepper to taste, and add paprika for color. Cover with foil and crimp the edges to form a seal. Bake at 450° for 20 minutes.
Servings: 4 proteins

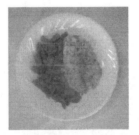

Rosemary Fish & Asparagus

100 grams white fish
 (ex. Orange Roughy, Tilapia, etc.) **Picture Q on back cover**
Italian Herb Seasoning grinder Fresh lemon juice
Rosemary grinder 2 c. asparagus
Ground pepper Garlic salt
Sea salt

Sprinkle both sides of fish with spices. Place fish on one side of preheated George Foreman grill. Top with a squeeze of fresh lemon juice. Place asparagus on the other side, sprinkled with garlic salt. Turn fish over after 2 minutes and give it another squeeze of lemon. Fish is done when flakes easily with a fork.
Servings: 1 protein, 1 vegetable

Spicy White Fish

100 grams white fish (ex. Orange Roughy, Tilapia, etc.)
Chili powder
Paprika
Garlic salt
Sea salt

Sprinkle both sides of fish with spices. Place on preheated
George Foreman grill. Turn over after 2 minutes. Fish is done
when flakes easily with a fork.
Servings: 1 protein

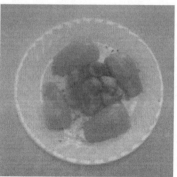

Sea Scallops with Fennel

Picture J on cover

1-2 heads fennel
1 T. apple cider vinegar
¾ t. fresh rosemary leaves or ¼ t. dried
4 drops Valencia Orange stevia
100 grams scallops
1 clove chopped garlic
Onion salt
Ground pepper

Cut fennel into quarters, remove core, and steam until tender
(about 15 minutes). Heat vinegar, rosemary, and stevia. Set
aside. Sauté scallops with chopped garlic over high heat until
lightly browned on both sides. Arrange scallops in center of
plate, surrounded with fennel. Sprinkle fennel with onion salt
and pepper. Pour vinegar sauce over scallops.
Servings: 1 protein, 1 vegetable

Boiled Lobster

Boiling is one of the easiest ways to prepare a lobster. Select a pot big enough to hold water to completely cover the lobsters. Bring the water to a rolling boil adding 1 tablespoon of salt per quart of water. Put the lobsters in with the claws first and start timing from the instant the water comes back to a boil.

Cooking time:
1 lb. - 5 minutes
1 1/8 lbs. - 6 minutes
1 1/4 lbs. - 8 minutes
1 1/2 to 2 lbs. - 8 to 10 minutes
more than 2 pounds : 12 minutes
Servings: 3 oz. cooked lobster = 1 protein

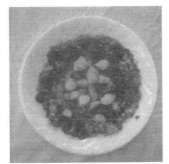

Seafood Gumbo   Picture P on cover

100 grams seafood (any combination of shrimp, scallops, lobster or white fish)

1 clove chopped garlic	1/8 t. garlic powder
2 large chopped Roma tomatoes	1/8 t. celery salt
¼ t. onion salt	1/8 t. ground cayenne pepper
¼ t. Creole seasoning	1-2 packets stevia

Sauté seafood with chopped garlic over high heat until lightly browned. Add remaining ingredients and simmer on low heat for 15 minutes.
Servings: 1 protein, 1 vegetable

Marinated Grilled Shrimp

110 grams large shrimp, peeled and deveined **with tails attached**

1½ t. chopped fresh parsley   1/8 t. salt
1 T. fresh lemon juice   1/8 t. ground black pepper
½ clove minced garlic   Skewers
¼ t. dried oregano

In a mixing bowl, mix together parsley, lemon juice, garlic, oregano, salt, and black pepper. Pour marinade into a small resealable plastic bag with shrimp. Seal, and marinate in the refrigerator for 2 hours. Preheat grill for medium-low heat. Thread shrimp onto skewers, piercing once near the tail and once near the head. Cook shrimp for 5 minutes per side, or until opaque.
Servings: 1 protein

Vegetable Steamed Lobster

1 T. salt per 1 quart water added
1 2 lb. Maine lobster
½ roughly chopped medium onion
1 roughly chopped stalk celery
½ t. cracked peppercorns
1 bay leaf
whole branches of fresh dill (if no dill, substitute tarragon or parsley)

Cover vegetables and seasonings with 1½ inches of water and bring to a boil. The vegetables will not be eaten, just used to make the lobster flavorful. Add the steamer basket with the lobster in it and cover tightly. Cook for 15 minutes, making sure there's still enough water in the bottom of the pot. If you do add more water, it is not necessary to add more salt, because only the water evaporates. Check for doneness with one of the small legs. After removing from the pot, weigh out 3 oz. of lobster for the HCG dieter and enjoy!
Servings: 3 proteins

Grilled Rock Lobster

1 t. salt
1 t. paprika
1/8 t. white pepper
1/8 t. garlic powder
2 T. water
2 T. fresh lemon juice
2 10 oz. thawed rock lobster tails

Split rock tails lengthwise with a large knife. Mix seasoning
with lemon juice and water. Brush meat side of tail with
marinade. Pre-heat grill and place rock tails meat side down and
grill five to six minutes until well scored. Turn over lobster and
cook another six minutes, brushing often with remaining
marinade.   Lobster is done when it is opaque and firm to the
touch.
Servings: 3 oz. cooked lobster = 1 protein

Italian Dill Fillets

4 100 gram pieces of fish (Orange Roughy, Pullock, Tilapia, etc.)
½ c. Vinaigrette dressing (pg. 13)
1 t. dried dill weed

Preheat oven to 400. Pour the vinaigrette into a measuring cup.
Stir in the dill. Arrange the fillets in 1 layer in a 13 x 9 inch
baking dish. Pour the sauce over the fish and bake, uncovered,
until the fish is opaque throughout and flakes easily with a fork,
8-12 minutes. Carefully place a fillet on each serving plate,
spoon some of the dressing over the fish, and serve at once.
Servings: 4 proteins

Garlic Shrimp

3/4 lb. small shrimp in their shells
Salt
Paprika, preferably Spanish
4 T. Chicken Bouillon Base (pg. 20)
4 sliced garlic cloves
¼ t. crushed red pepper flakes
1 T. fresh lemon juice
2 T. minced parsley

Shell the shrimp and sprinkle with salt and paprika. Heat the bouillon base, garlic and pepper flakes in a medium skillet. When the garlic is just beginning to brown, add the shrimp and cook, stirring, about 1 minute, or until just done and firm to the touch. Stir in the lemon juice, and parsley. Serve immediately.
Servings: 3 oz. cooked shrimp = 1 protein

Orange Roughy with Orange Sauce Recipe

½ lb. orange roughy fillets
1/3 t. stemmed fresh lemon thyme or any thyme
1 T. water
2 chopped red onions
1 orange, sectioned, peel thinly sliced
1/3 bunch stemmed fresh cilantro
1/8 t. salt

Rinse fish and pat dry. Pat thyme on both sides, set aside. Heat water in nonstick skillet over medium high heat. Add half of the onion and salt and cook, stirring, until onions are soft (3-4 minutes).

Add fish, reduce heat to medium and cover pan. Cook until fish flakes easily (6-8 minutes). Toss remaining onion, orange sections, peel, cilantro and salt and serve over cooked fish. Dividing recipe in half yields an HCG dieter 1 protein, 1 vegetable and ½ fruit.
Servings: 2 proteins, 2 vegetables, 1 fruit

Greek Red Snapper

1 large Snapper, cleaned and scaled, heads on or off
2 T. water
1 t. oregano
1 t. salt
5 T. fresh lemon juice
1/3 t. pepper
1 crushed garlic clove
Dash of paprika

Place the fish in foil and broil for 5 minutes, then turn. Cook another 3 minutes.
In a bowl mix all ingredients. Brush fish every 3 minutes, or until done, approximately 30-35 minutes. Take out and sprinkle with lemon juice.
Servings: 3 oz. cooked fish = 1 protein

Venison Entrees

Since venison (deer) is a wild meat, we imagine Dr. Simeons most probably did not use venison in his experiments with the diet. With being much leaner than beef, we have had many clients use venison during the 500 calorie phase with very good results, so we have included some venison recipes.

South of the Border Venison Steaks

2 100 gram pieces venison   1 ½ t. All-Purpose Seasoning (pg. 15)
¾ t. fresh lemon juice   ¾ t. chili powder
¾ t. chopped fresh cilantro

Combine lemon juice with chopped cilantro. Mix together steak seasoning and chili powder in a small bowl. Rub the seasoning blend onto both sides of the steaks. Grill on med-high heat for 5 to 8 minutes on each side to achieve medium doneness. To serve, transfer to serving dish and top with juice mixture.
Servings: 2 proteins

Marinated Venison Steaks

4 100 gram lean venison steaks
3 T. Chicken Bouillon Base (pg. 20)
¼ c. water   1 t. fresh rosemary
½ t. minced garlic   1/8 t. ground cumin
1/8 t. cayenne pepper   1/8 t. paprika
1 T. apple cider vinegar   Sea salt
2 t. chopped fresh parsley   Pepper
½ leaf chopped fresh basil

Combine water, Chicken Bouillon Base, garlic and cayenne pepper in a saucepan and bring to a boil. Reduce heat and stir in vinegar, parsley, basil, rosemary, cumin, paprika, salt and pepper. Simmer for 20 minutes, stirring frequently. Remove from heat. Pour cooled mixture over venison steaks in a sealable bag and marinate in the refrigerator for 4 hours turning regularly. Take steaks out of bag, reserving marinade. Grill steaks on high heat for about 7 minutes on each side. Make sure not to overcook. Baste steaks with left-over marinade while grilling.
Servings: 4 proteins

Shopping List

Herbs, Spices, Seasonings

Allspice
Apple Cider Vinegar
Basil
Bay Leaf
Cayenne Pepper
Celery Salt
Chili Powder
Chili Seasoning
Chinese Style Five Spice
Cilantro (fresh)
Cinnamon
Coriander
Creole Seasoning
Cumin (ground)
Dill (fresh)
Dill Seed
Garlic Cloves
Garlic Granules
Garlic Powder
Garlic Salt
Ginger
Ground Black Pepper

Italian Seasoning
McCormick Italian Seasoning
Mint Leaves (dried or fresh)
Nutmeg
Onion Powder
Onion Salt
Oregano (dried)
Paprika
Parsley (fresh or dried)
Peppercorns
Poultry Seasoning
Rosemary (fresh or dried)
Sage (Dried)
Sea Salt
Seasonings/Spices/Herbs
Thyme
Thyme Leaves
Tony Chacherc's Original Creole Seasoning
Turmeric
White Pepper

Vegetables

Asparagus
Beet Greens
Cabbage
Celery Chard
Cucumber

Fennel
Lettuce (i.e. Romaine)
Onion (i.e. Vidalia)
Radishes
Spinach

Tomatoes (Regular, Roma, Grape)

Fruits

Apples
Grapefruits
Lemons

Oranges
Strawberries

Miscellaneous

Grissino
Melba Toast

Stevia

Liquid Stevia Flavors:

Apricot Nectar Stevia

Chocolate Raspberry Stevia

Chocolate Stevia

Cinnamon Stevia

Clear Liquid Stevia

English Toffee Stevia

Grape Stevia

Lemon Stevia

Orange Valencia

Root Beer Stevia

Vanilla Cream Stevia

Packets of Stevia i.e. Only Sweet or SweetLeaf

Beverages

Carbonated Water

Coffee

Milk

Meat

Beef Steak (lean i.e. Sirloin)

Beef, Ground (93% or better Fat-Free)

Chicken Breast

Veal

Fish and Seafood

Crab (NOT imitation)

Crab Legs

Fish (Orange Roughy, Tilapia, Flounder, Chilean Sea Bass, Red Snapper)

Lobster

Scallops

Shrimp

The following excerpts are given with express written permission from the author of the HCG Weight Loss Cure Guide (available on Amazon.com).

Most Common Errors during 500 Calorie Diet Phase

1. Not loading enough fat during load days (first two days of HCG). This might explain hunger and associated crankiness during the first week of HCG low calorie phase.

2. Mixing vegetables at a meal. Dr. Simeons clearly states one vegetable. While many people lose quite satisfactorily when mixing vegetables, it is a place to review if losing slows.

3. No gum, mints, etc. allowed during the VLCD (very low calorie diet phase). Again, some lose quite satisfactorily when violating this directive, but it is a place to review if losing slows.

4. No diet drinks including Crystal Light, diet soda or other diet drinks – only water, teas, coffees, and mineral water. Remember, you get one lemon to use each day.

5. American beef is noted as significantly more fatty than the beef Dr. Simeons refers to. Veal is a suggested replacement, but veal is only carried locally at Dierburgs (St. Louis, MO area) to our knowledge at this time. Buffalo is less fatty than American beef and is available at Trader Joe's at this time. Many participants can quicken weight loss by eating less beef and more chicken or allowable fish/seafood, in particular.

6. Weight of protein is to be based on PRECOOKED weight, not post cooking – this can make quite a difference in the prescribed serving with certain proteins.

7. Eating the same protein for both lunch and dinner. Food selections are to be varied.

8. Not drinking enough water – you should be drinking at least 2 quarts of allowable liquids per day.

9. Try to weigh in the same clothes or something very similar in weight and around the same time each morning (before eating or drinking) in order to avoid confusion or false appearance of weight gain/loss.

10. Avoid eating at restaurants because to a large degree the meats have been 'juiced' or manipulated to be more flavorful, tender or juicy with a multitude of processes that could easily slow your weight loss, particularly chicken.

Time Saving Tips

➤ Purchase thawed protein servings (shrimp, chicken breast, crab, and fish) and, instead of putting it in the freezer in big quantities, divide the portions into the prescribed 100 gram servings, then freeze in individual size servings. Note: Some participants take this one step further and actually cook the protein before freezing so that it can just be reheated or put on a salad before eating.

➤ Each morning (or the night before) pick two different proteins for the upcoming day and move them to the refrigerator to thaw. Thawing won't take long and cooking only takes a couple of minutes on the George Foreman grill. This saves very much time compared to putting blocks of frozen chicken breasts, etc. and trying to work with it when you want your 100 grams for a meal.

➤ Fill 7-14 syringes at a time instead of one every morning.

➤ Grissino breadsticks can be found at Schnucks in the deli/cheese area.

➤ Melba toast can be found at Wal-Mart, Shop N Save, and other stores, but it can be a little tricky to locate. Sometimes it is near crackers, other times it may be in the salad dressing/crouton area.

➤ Use a George Foreman grill for meat – almost everything is done in about 3 minutes.

Plateau Breakers and Daily Loss Rate Maximizers

➤ Increase water intake to 2 - 3 quarts per day.

➤ Try adding a glass or two of green tea to your day.

➤ Don't eat 2 apples for the two fruits or cut down on the size of the apples.

➤ Cut American beef down or out.

➤ Check all condiments for any form of sugar. 'Garlic Salt' may list sugar as an ingredient. Any seasoning salt or seasoning product must be carefully checked.

➤ If mixing vegetables, stop.

➤ If having trouble with constipation, try Smooth Move tea – most people find this to be very effective. Check in the specialty tea section of grocery store or a local health food store.

➤ Try leaving out one or both breadsticks.

These plateau breakers/rate loss maximizers and many more ideas are listed in the HCG Weight Loss Cure Guide (available at PoundsAndInchesAway.com and Amazon.com).

Best Advice...Be Intentional...A Philosophy of Sorts

When beginning an HCG diet protocol, we find it imperative to impress upon clients the requirement to BE INTENTIONAL. This applies to everything you eat and everything that comes in contact with your skin.

While we followed Dr. Simeons protocol (Pounds and Inches), there are other HCG protocols that differ —some to a slight degree and others to a large degree. Dr. Simeons worked on his protocol for about 40 years, so we feel confident that he knew EXACTLY what he was talking about. So, for example, when someone says, "Well, green beans and broccoli are really good for you AND every other diet lets you have those, so why can't we have those?" or "Do you really think they will hurt anything?" OR, my personal all-time favorite, "I ate them and they didn't make any difference!"...My response is "I guarantee you that Dr. Simeons didn't just forget about green beans and broccoli, only to remember beet greens and fennel. I guarantee he tried them, and that the results were simply not as favorable." In summary, no one knows for sure that bending the rules did NOT 'hurt' them. For example, if they mixed vegetables or ate un-allowed vegetables, or did other slight variances, a person doesn't know how much they would have lost if they had NOT mixed vegetables or NOT had green beans or NOT had a seasoning spice that contained sugar or starch in some, small form.

We have seen many people stall due to seasonings. You must realize that something as harmless as garlic salt may have several ingredients that potentially stall you -- even just a few sprinkles. It is a common occurrence for us to have clients get all of their spices out at one time and read us all ingredients – not the food nutritional values; but the actual ingredients. When one person stalled she reported only using salt, pepper, and garlic salt. The problem was that the 'innocent' garlic salt had both sugar and modified corn starch listed as ingredients. If you think this can't stall you, we have found differently. So, with regard to spice – BE INTENTIONAL.

If your hands are extremely dry – BE INTENTIONAL. That might mean trying to get by without your typical hand lotion, then trying to get by with just mineral oil, ; however, at some point before you actually bleed, you may have to put a slight healing lotion on your hands twice a day vs. slathering on 10 times a day, etc. – BE INTENTIONAL.

The same 'dry' situation can occur to your lips. I have very sparsely applied medicated Blistex to my lips once or twice during a cycle. This is instead of putting ointment on my lips about 10 times a day – BE INTENTIONAL.

If your George Foreman grill is starting to stick to meat and/or vegetables, you may decide to spray the grill with nonstick cooking spray. Be aware that ¼ of a second is a 'serving' and that it doesn't take many sprays to add some nutritional value to your food. So, BE INTENTIONAL and spray very quickly.

Eating out while on the protocol isn't easy, but it is necessary sometimes. One meal I have consistently lost weight after is McDonald's grilled chicken Caesar salad. I take off the cheese and carrots as best I can and, obviously, don't use the crouton pack. I either bring my own dressing or sprinkle my salad with a little stevia sweetened, iced tea—my way of BEING INTENTIONAL. Never throw in the towel while HCG is pulsing through your system – you can simply gain too easily.

One client had an ear blockage for which her doctor prescribed an oil based ear drop. With just a few drops, she gained 3 pounds – we know it doesn't make sense with our common knowledge, but it also doesn't matter that it doesn't make sense. Her condition had been building for some time and did not require immediate treatment, so she stopped the oil until she was done with her current HCG cycle – BE INTENTIONAL. (P.S. She did proceed with her treatment after the cycle and, of course, did not gain weight because the HCG was then out of her system.)

You will find several people who boast about losing weight while cheating, mixing vegetables, using un-allowed spices, having salsa, drinking alcohol here and there, etc. While they have continued to lose, please always remember that it only means that they could have possibly lost more AND that they may be bypassing the opportunity for resetting their metabolism to the fullest extent possible, thereby jeopardizing their future weight maintenance capabilities. So, minimize stretching or compromising any rules, in any way, for medical, social or other reasons—ALWAYS BE INTENTIONAL in order to maximize the overall effect on your incredible weight loss journey.

About the Authors

Rest assured, both authors (biological sisters) have successfully completed at least 2 rounds of HCG dieting.

Leanne has lost over 45 pounds, is the mother of 9 children, and is wearing a size 8 for the first time in her LIFE.

Linda has lost about 30 pounds, is the mother of 8 children, and is also a size 8 for the first time in her LIFE.

Even more importantly, both are maintaining the loss. Additionally, the authors have experience in helping many friends, relatives and clients –some through multiple 'cycles'. Success both during the diet phase and afterwards has been fun, exciting and impressive. On average, clients lose 20 – 30 pounds in a cycle.

These results ARE typical!!!

Consulting with many clients on the diet continues to provide helpful learning experiences and new recipes here and there. Check out the website occasionally as new information will continue to be added. Best wishes to everyone who takes on this exciting journey!